Feed the Body and Soul

Feed the Body and Soul

FOOD AND YOGA FOR EVERY SEASON

• • •

Arianna Sertoli

ISBN: 1530230705
ISBN 13: 9781530230709

Library of Congress Control Number: 2016907772
CreateSpace Independent Publishing Platform
North Charleston, South Carolina

I dedicate this book to my father, whose diagnosis and treatment of colon cancer invigorated my curiosity to discover more about the path to a holistic self-care and the benefit of healthy eating. When my father, an important pillar of my life, passed, I became the woman I am today.

Contents

CHAPTER 1
A Little Introduction

• • •

IF YOU PICKED UP THIS book, you're curious, as I was, to understand the importance of a balanced, clean, and happy life. This book is an integration of feeding the body with delicious and healthy foods and feeding the soul with yoga poses, all focused around the different seasons. I want to bring back the true meaning of cooking at home, and I want to focus on how simple and delicious your food can be without too much work. Eating real, whole, in-season food is simple. We need to go back to what our grandmothers used to do and not rely on packaged, microwavable, factory-farmed, manufactured, and fast foods. In today's world people don't have time to spend on cooking elaborate meals, and when they get home, all they want is to put something on the table that tastes good and is simple. If that describes you, then here is the perfect book!

As for yoga, you don't have to be a yogi to simply practice a few movements daily to make your body and mind de-stress and to release tension. I have chosen four poses to help you gain some balance during the different times of the year. When I am on the mat, I feel I am in a safe place, and I can dedicate that time to myself. Remember, if you feel good, your energy will be stronger, and people will see your happiness and glow.

Now a little history on how I came to love food and yoga. I spent my first year of life in Bhutan and was introduced to their spices and different foods. When I was growing up, my father loved Japanese food—salty mocha, miso soup, seaweed, and plum vinegar were all things we ate regularly. I believe that introductions to different flavors when you are little teach you to be always curious to try new things.

Later on I remember going to the farmers' market with my mother and cooking with her in the kitchen; she was a self-taught cook, and she passed on to me a love for the kitchen, making me want to discover more. Healthy foods were always in my life, and the dining table was filled with seasonal vegetables, fruits, healthy proteins, and not many packaged foods.

In 2012 my father was diagnosed with colon cancer, and while taking care of him, I tried to learn more about food and its importance in recovery. After his death I decided I wanted to know even more, and I enrolled in the Integrative Institute of Nutrition, while at the same time pursuing yoga-teacher training. These two decisions have been the best my life. Today I love spreading the knowledge of how to have a healthy life and be happy.

At the time that I was taking care of my father, I was diagnosed with Hashimoto's disease (a condition where your immune system attacks your thyroid), and I was able to reverse it by simply tweaking my diet, practicing meditation and yoga, and learning how to de-stress.

Food is made out of fire, water, air, and earth elements, and these keep us alive. Remember that we are what we eat. Embracing this concept, I believe food is one of the most important tools we have to keep ourselves healthy and strong. I also know that the ingredients need to be clean; this means no genetically modified crops, factory-farmed meat, or unknown ingredients in your food. Choose food that is produced with love and care. Keep your food clean and grown with love, and I promise it will taste delicious.

I love to try new recipes to understand how different ingredients work with each other. I want to spread this happiness to the world through this book.

Now let's get in the kitchen! And later, let's practice our yoga positions.

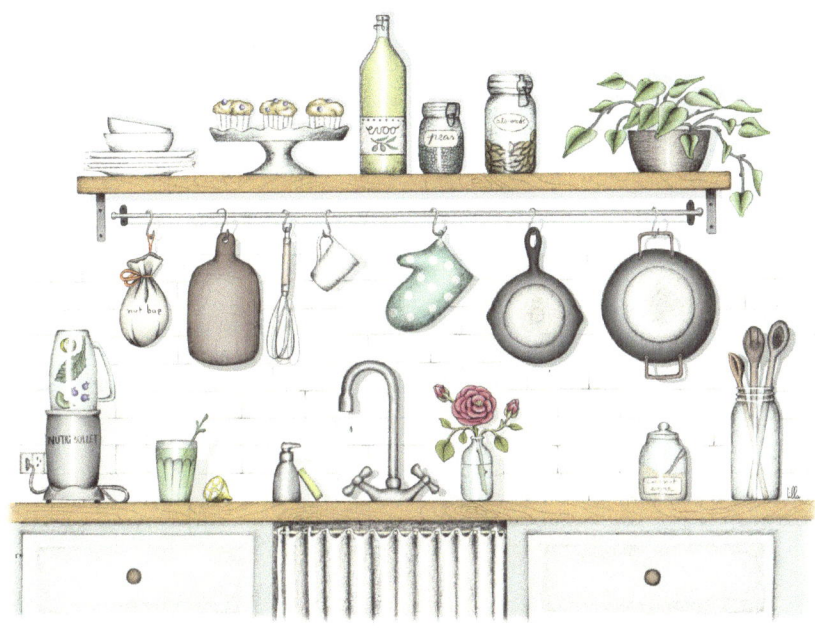

CHAPTER 2

Kitchen and Pantry Essentials

• • •

MUST-HAVES IN THE KITCHEN

THIS LIST CONTAINS EVERYTHING I believe you should have in the kitchen to keep your eating clean and your kitchen free of chemicals.

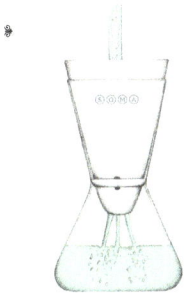

- Water filters: There are many different filters available in the market, and the choices can range in price from a few dollars to thousands. I believe in getting something in the medium range to ensure quality without breaking the bank. My top choice is the Soma. This water pitcher is made of unbreakable glass instead of plastic. The filters are biodegradable and are made with coconut shells that are heat treated to create a natural, highly absorbent carbon filter. Soma will deliver their filters to your home for your convenience.

- GreenPan cookware: It's now pretty common knowledge that Teflon is dangerous for your health. It's time for a change. My favorite pans and pots are GreenPan Thermolon nonstick ceramic pans, heavy-bottomed pots (perfect for stews), cast-iron skillets (perfect for making quiches and oven eggs), and stainless-steel pots and pans (a chef's favorite because of stainless steel's great conductivity and long life-span).

* Blender: A blender is a must-have in your kitchen to make soups, smoothies, nondairy milks, sauces, dips, and so much more. The choices are wide; once again you can go from fairly inexpensive to pricey. I use the NutriBullet, which offers many different containers that work perfectly for a variety of uses.

* 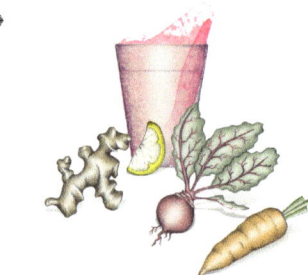 Cold-press juicer: This juicer is a great way to save money on your green juice; make it yourself instead! There are many good juicers on the market. Make sure the one you get is a cold-press one; the other ones warm up the juice and kill all the minerals and vitamins the vegetables and fruits contain. A tip for juicing is to use the least amount of fruits possible, in order to not add unnecessary sugar to your diet, and to keep your juices simple and organic as much as possible.

* Nut bag: Another way to save money and avoid additives in your nut milk is to make it yourself. Any nut milk is very simple to make and will have no extra additives such as carrageenan, soy lecithin, or sugar.

* 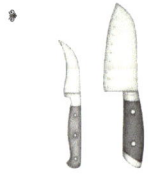 Wooden cookware: Plastic is a bit controversial because of its health-related issues; as an Italian I love wooden spoons that can be used for almost every cooking scenario, and they are made in various sizes and shapes, depending on your needs. Also, they won't scratch your pans.

* Glass jars: Buying in bulk is the best way to avoid boxed food with extra additives and to save money. Having glass jars will allow you to put grains, beans, and other bulk food items in reach as you need them and will keep the pantry clean and effective.

* Good-quality knives: I have a wide collection of knives, and each one has a specific purpose. The knives' quality needs to be good, and knives need good care. A chef's knife will be your main cutting utensil; a ceramic knife and a Japanese knife can be used if you want to explore your cutting skills. Make sure you sharpen them a few times a week, clean them with cold water, and dry them right away.

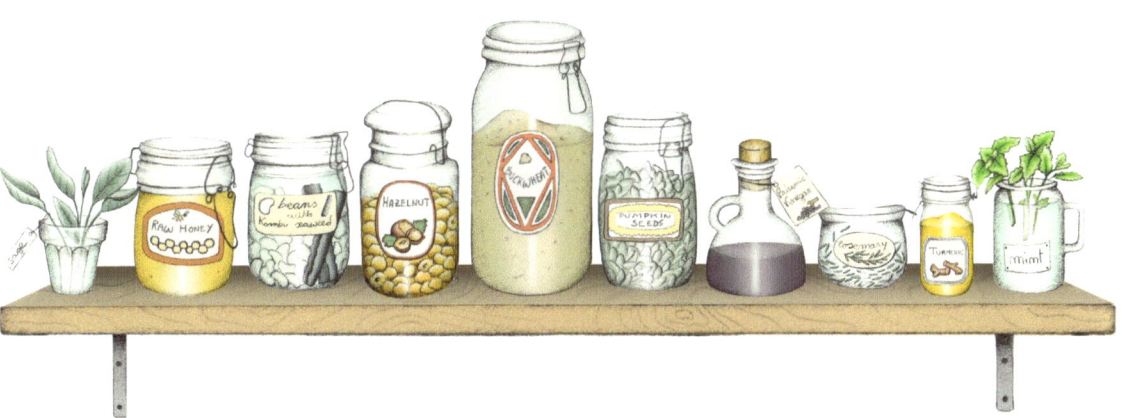

MUST-HAVES IN THE PANTRY

There are some staples you want to always have in the kitchen to give food extra flavor. These will also give you options for healthy meals when there is nothing in the fridge.

- Nuts and seeds: These are perfect for your salads, desserts, trail mixes, and soups. They are full of good fats, omega-3s, and energy boosters. Buy raw ones, possibly organic, and make both nut butters and milks with them; they are very easy to make. Seed options include flax, chia, sesame, hemp, pumpkin, and sunflower; nut options include macadamia, almond, walnut, pistachio, pine nut, brazil nut, cashew, and hazelnut.

- Gluten-free grains: Many people today are gluten intolerant or have celiac disease, but there are many healthy grains that they can still eat, such as quinoa, millet, buckwheat, rice, and amaranth. Oats are not always gluten-free, so make sure you check before buying them. Before cooking, soak buckwheat, quinoa, or rice in some water with kombu seaweed to break down the phytic acid and saponins that make them harder to digest. Some of these grains also come as pastas, soba, or various Japanese noodles to spice things up in the kitchen.

- Beans and lentils: Buy these in bulk; they are pretty simple to make. Just soak the beans in water with possibly some kombu seaweed to break down the antinutrients, such as phytic acid and enzyme inhibitor (which make you gassy and give you heartburn, reflux, and bloating). Lentils don't need to be soaked, and they cook faster.

- Oils: Extra virgin olive, sesame, macadamia, coconut, walnut, hemp, and flax oils are some of the top oils to use for cooking and dressings because of their healthy fats, taste, and cooking ability. Stick as much as possible with organic oils, and avoid mixed and vegetable oil ones such as canola or safflower.

- Vinegars: Your food can go to a whole new level when you add a little extra kick in the form of vinegar. I use mainly balsamic, apple cider, plum, or rice wine.

- Natural sweeteners: Ditch the sugar—it's just a high-glycemic element that your body doesn't need and that is completely deadly for you. Instead, use natural sweeteners such as maple syrup, dried fruits (e.g., dates, prunes, figs, and apricots), coconut sugar, or raw and local honey. They taste delicious, and your body will feel so much better afterward.

- Herbs and spices: Being Italian I use fresh herbs a lot. If you have space on your terrace or in your kitchen window, plant some basil, thyme, sage, mint, oregano, and rosemary. If not, buy a bunch, and then, to keep it fresh, put it in water in the fridge. It will last longer. Spices are another great source to make your food even tastier and fancier. Many of these have health benefits, from being anti-inflammatory to helping cleanse your body from extra toxins. Keep your spice rack full, and stick with organic.

- Butter and ghee from grass-fed cows: Butter was controversial for a while, but after the *New York Times* article "Butter is Back" in 2014, we understand that a little bit of fresh butter from a grass-fed cow, sheeps, or goats is OK. Obviously it is not an item to indulge in, but at times it might give extra flavor to your food. Ghee is clarified butter, which is more easily digested and lighter.

CHAPTER 3

Dirty Dozen and Clean Fifteen

• • •

THE ENVIRONMENTAL WORKING GROUP DESIGNED one guide for produce that should always be bought organic or at the farmers' market because of high pesticide content and another guide for vegetables and fruits that are fine to buy conventionally. Try to buy vegetables as clean as possible.

DIRTY DOZEN (MUST BUY ORGANIC)

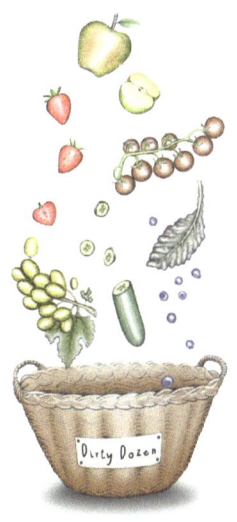

- Celery
- Spinach
- Sweet bell peppers
- Nectarines (imported)
- Cucumbers
- Cherry tomatoes
- Strawberries
- Grapes
- Snap peas (imported)
- White potatoes
- Strawberries
- Grapes
- Snap peas (imported)
- White Potatoes

Extra

- Hot peppers
- Blueberries (domestic)
- Zucchini

CLEAN FIFTEEN (OK TO BUY CONVENTIONAL)

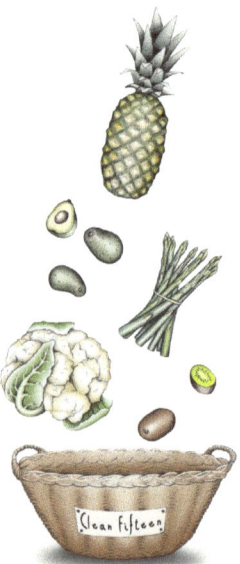

- Avocados
- Sweet corn
- Pineapples
- Cabbage
- Sweet peas (frozen)
- Onions
- Asparagus
- Mangoes
- Papayas
- Kiwi
- Eggplant
- Grapefruit
- Cantaloupe (domestic)
- Cauliflower
- Sweet potatoes

CHAPTER 4
Five Food Rules

• • •

1. Eat slow, and chew a lot.

Today we eat fast because we say that we have no time, but I believe this is not a good excuse. Our bodies need proper nutrition, and the nutrition needs to be digested properly to help the body take full advantage of it. When you have your plate in front of you, don't just shovel your food into your mouth; savor it by eating slowly, maybe putting down your fork between every few bites. If you want to fill up and maybe lose those extra pounds, here is a good tip that works: chew until the food gets liquefied. The digestion process starts in the mouth—don't make the stomach and intestines do all the work.

2. Drink warmer water, and not during meals.

Drink room-temperature water fifteen to twenty minutes before or after food. Your body needs water and hydration, since 60 percent of it is made up of water. In the United States, ice is routinely added to water, which makes the stomach work to warm it up instead of focusing on the digestion process; this slows down the whole digestion process. Ask for water with no ice at restaurants, and you will feel the difference.

Also consider not drinking during eating, because this interferes with your saliva, enzymes, and stomach acid and makes it harder for your digestive track to break down your food. If you drink before or after a meal instead, you will feel more satisfied and fuller, and you will help the body get the right hydration.

3. Eat consciously.

Today we forget the importance of eating; it's not only about feeding the body and scarfing food down your throat. Give your food a chance, and try to eat consciously by realizing what you are putting in your body, chewing slowly, and not just rushing through the meal.

4. SIT AT A TABLE (WITH FAMILY OR FRIENDS OR AWAY FROM THE COMPUTER AND PHONE).

Electronic devices are becoming more a part of our everyday lives, making us forget to give our bodies some time off from computers and phones when eating. Try to get to the lunchroom, and sit at a dining table; maybe get a magazine if alone, or sit with people and have some human contact. It will make you appreciate life and food more. In Italy, families sit together at dinner every night or have a family lunch on Sundays to remember the importance of being all together.

5. MAKE YOUR FOOD WITH LOVE.

Vitamin "love" is one of the most important vitamins in our lives, and it is not only about the relationship with your significant other, friend, or cat but also about your relationship with food and the process of making it.

I love cooking—and if you picked up this book, you probably do too—so try to make food and spread love in the kitchen. Everyone at home will feel the different vibe, and you will too.

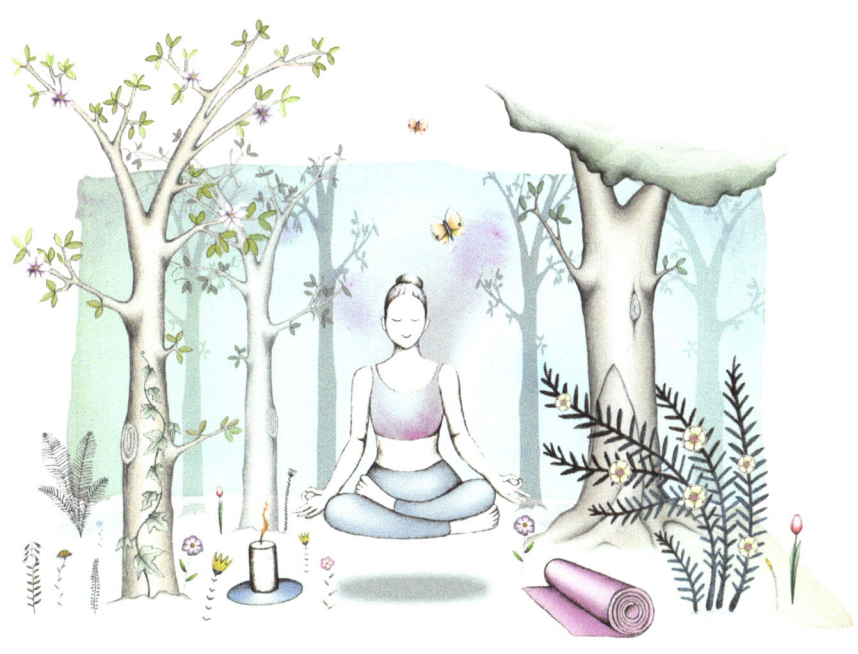

CHAPTER 5

Yoga Essentials

• • •

YOGA BENEFITS

YOGA COMES FROM VERY ANCIENT studies; it has been modified to benefit those living in today's world and culture. Studies have shown that yoga can help with recovery from injuries, autoimmune diseases, diabetes, obesity, and other health issues.

When I decided to dedicate myself to yoga, I noticed how I was able to build strength and learn to be calmer while keeping my body in shape.

Yoga is for all, and none need to become the next yogi of the year. Just have your own practice, and you will find your balance. Each yoga pose in this book was chosen based on the seasons and the benefits they provide because of them. Let's get started!

COMFORTABLE SPACE

When you decide to practice yoga, make sure you are in a calming and peaceful space. It can be your bedroom with a closed door, the park, a studio, or even your couch. You want to get everything that happened that day away from that space; make it a time for yourself. Remember, a yoga practice can be as long as several hours or as short as ten minutes.

BREATHE

The first step to start your practice is to breathe deeply. On your inhalation, feel your ribs expanding more than usual, close your eyes to make the experience a more sensorial one, and then take long exhalations. Keep breathing until you find your own rhythm and you get your mind calmed and settled.

LET GO!

When you decide to practice, even if vigorously, make sure you dedicate time to just relax, and take a couple of minutes in the final pose. Yoga is proven to de-stress the body and make the mind relax, especially after long days of work.

USEFUL TOOLS

You can use the floor, a blanket, or the carpet if you don't have a mat, but you can find organic mats at a good price everywhere now. Whether you are a beginner or a pro, don't hate your props, but use them. These can be a blanket for tight hips, legs, or sensitive knees; a block or book for allowing space into the body; the couch to stretch or back bend; and a belt to open legs, hips, or shoulders. Use what you need, and be gentle to yourself.

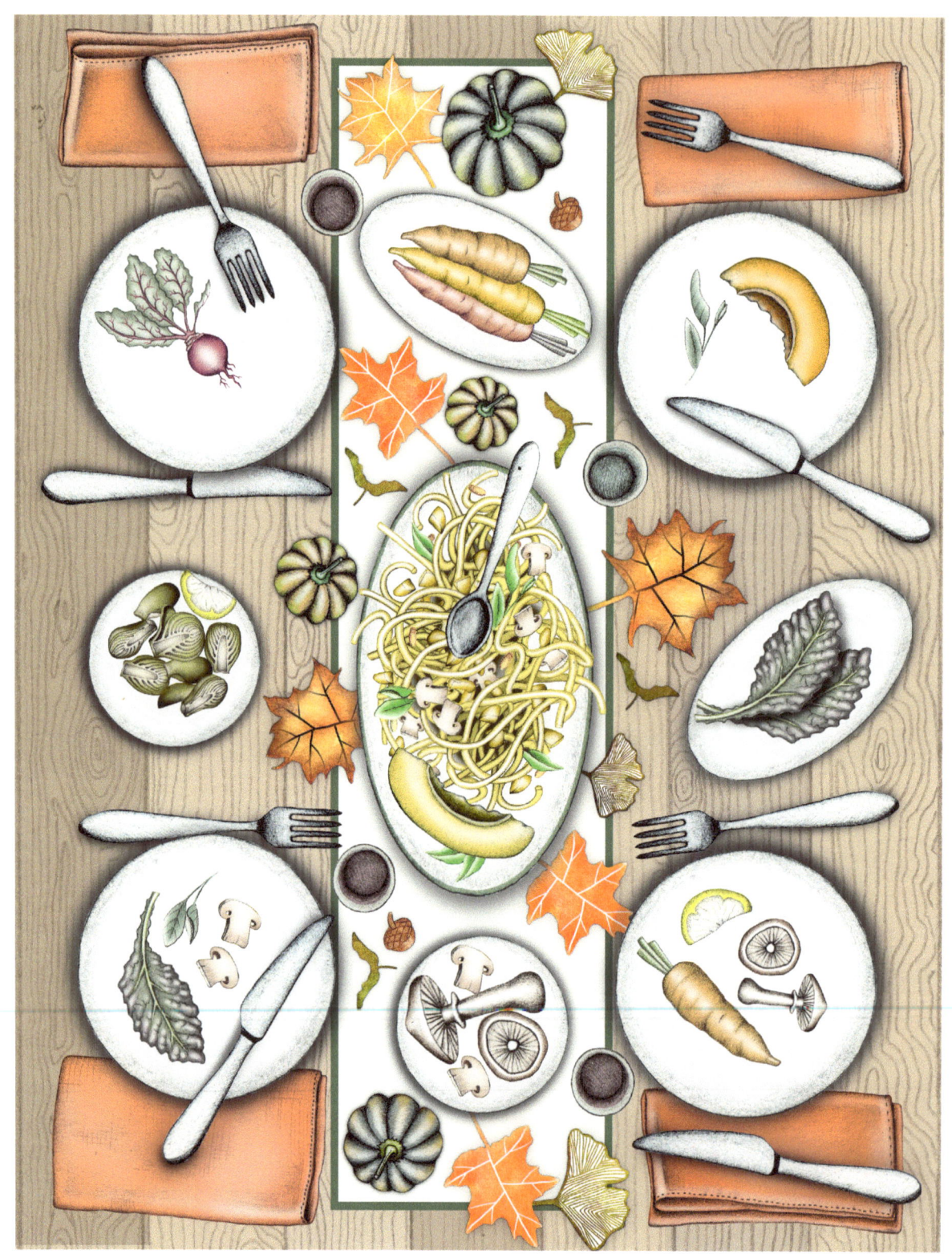

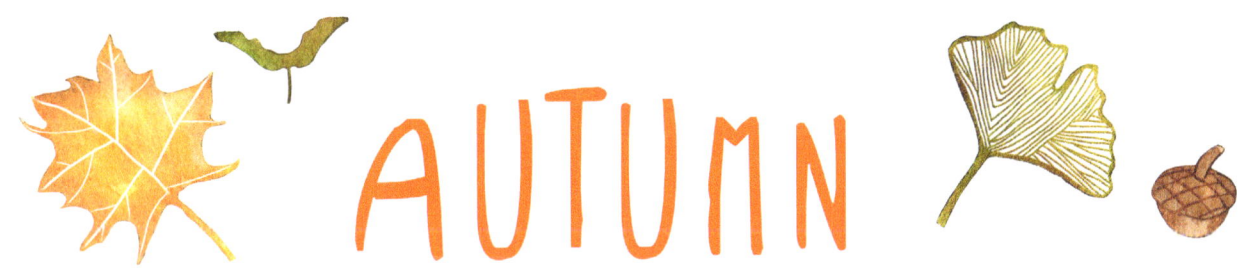

CHAPTER 6

Recipes and Yoga

• • •

Autumn is one of my favorite times of year. The leaves are falling; the weather is getting cooler. You still have that summer skin and memories, and slowly you start to be surrounded by shades of reds, oranges, and yellows. I love to make simple, warm foods this time of year.

In the fall, focus on harvest foods such as onions, sweet potatoes, and carrots to warm your soul. Be gentle, and include some warming spices such as ginger or peppercorn to embellish your food.

BRIDGE POSE (SETU BANDHA SARVANGASANA)

FALL IS THE TIME WHEN we need to go back to our regular routines. Try to make your practice a routine, too, to keep calm in this season of change.

Bridge pose brings energy to your spine, as you root your feet into the ground. It is a great pose to reduce anxiety, fatigue, insomnia, and backache, and it stimulates important organs such as the lungs and thyroid. It is also a very good pose for releasing menstrual back pains.

This position can be modified with a block under the sacrum to make it more relaxing.

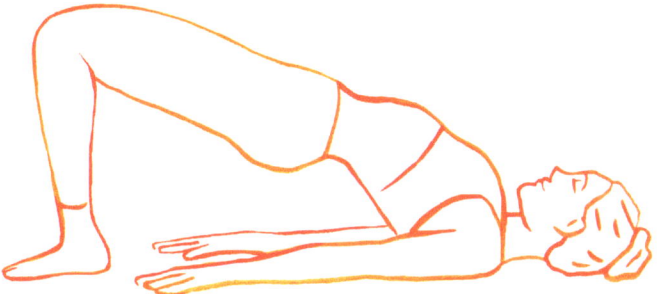

BREAKFAST

APPLE BLUEBERRY OATMEAL PIE

Serves 4

1 apple
1½ cups blueberries
2 cups oatmeal

1 cup almond meal
honey or maple syrup, to taste
olive oil, to taste

Preheat the oven to 350°F. Cut the apple into half-moons and set in an oven pan; in the center of the pan, add the blueberries. In a separate bowl, add oatmeal, almond meal, sweetener of choice, and olive oil, and mix well with a wooden spoon or hands. Set the mixture on top of the fruit. Bake for twenty minutes or until the top is browned.

LUNCH

SEASONAL VEGGIES AND MILLET

Serves 2

1 cup millet	1 cup sliced mushrooms
1 piece kombu seaweed	1 cup kale, chopped small
1½ cups water, for cooking	1 large carrot, cubed
1 garlic clove, minced	salt
pepitas	balsamic vinegar
olive oil	parsley, to garnish

Soak the millet and kombu in water for a minimum of twenty minutes. Rinse. In a saucepan, add the grains to one and one-half cups of water, and bring to a boil. Add one teaspoon of salt; cover and cook for fifteen minutes at low heat until the water is completely absorbed.

In a pan, add some olive oil and the garlic, and roast for a few seconds. Add the carrots first with a tiny bit of water; cover and cook for five minutes. When they are almost soft, add the mushrooms and brown. Finally add the kale, pepitas, and vinegar. When the millet is ready, toss with the vegetables, and add the chopped parsley.

PEAR AND WALNUT SALAD

Serves 4

2 pears	balsamic vinegar
3 walnuts	olive oil
3 cups arugula	salt, to taste

Cut the pears into slices, chop the walnuts into halves, and then toss everything with some arugula. In a separate cup, mix the condiments together; pour it onto the salad, mix it all up, and serve. It's a refreshing meal on a warmer autumn day.

Roasted Brussels Sprouts with Amaranth and Lemon Sauce

Serves 2

1½ cups amaranth

½ lemon

2 cups brussels sprouts

1 teaspoon raw honey

olive oil

salt, to taste

1 white onion

2 tablespoons lukewarm water

Cook the amaranth at a one-to-one ratio of grain and water. Preheat the oven to 350°F. Cut the brussels sprouts in half, and set in a pan with a tiny bit of water; cover and cook on medium heat for ten minutes, until almost fully ready. Drain the excess water, and set in the oven for another ten minutes. Finely chop the onion. In a pan, add some olive oil, and cook the onion until soft.

In a small bowl, mix olive oil, salt, honey, and water, and stir quickly to make the dressing. When the amaranth is ready, add the onion and brussels sprouts, and cover with the sauce.

Snack

Pumpkin Energy Balls

Serves 4

1 cup pitted dates

1 tablespoon sliced almonds

1 cup lukewarm water

¾ cup pumpkin puree

Toppings:

1 teaspoon ginger powder

shredded coconut

1 tablespoon pumpkin seeds

raw cocoa

1 tablespoon hemp seeds

chia seeds

Set the pitted dates in the lukewarm water for two minutes to soften. Put all the other ingredients in the blender, and add the dates. Mix for four minutes, until it becomes a hard mixture, and with your hands make small balls and place on a plate; sprinkle with topping of choice. This will give you energy during that afternoon slump when the vending machine, sugar-loaded snacks look so appealing.

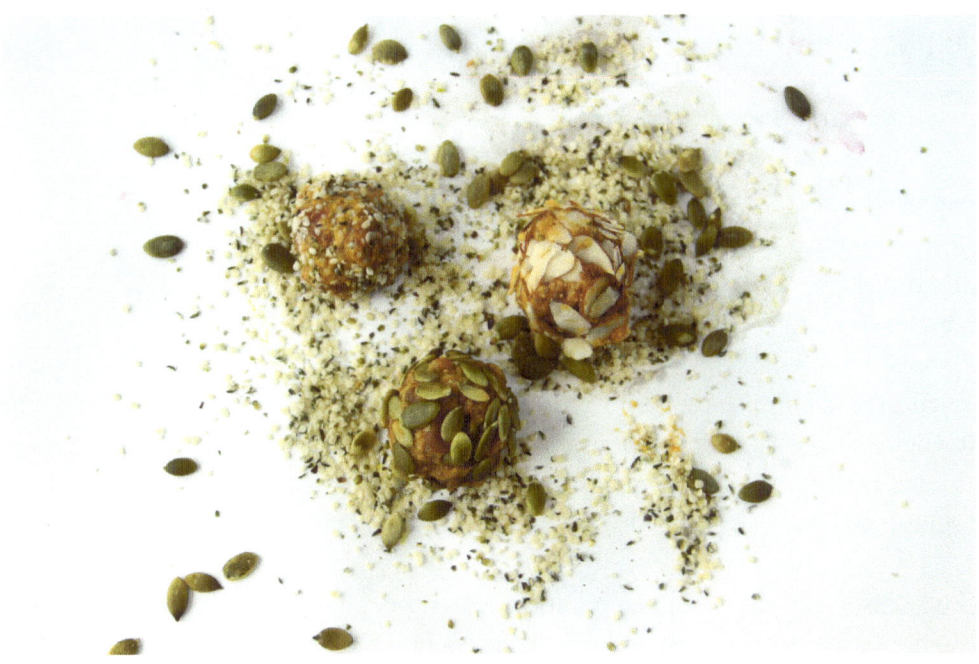

DINNER

ROASTED TURKEY BREAST WITH GRAVY

Serves 2

2 organic turkey breasts
olive oil
salt
pepper
1 teaspoon kuzu
1 teaspoon mirin

1 tablespoon fresh sage
1 tablespoon rice vinegar
5 sprigs of juniper

In a ceramic pan, add some olive oil. When the pan is warm, add the turkey breast and sauté until it reaches a firmer state.

In a small saucepan, add all the other ingredients and salt to taste. Heat at a low flame for ten to fifteen minutes, stirring, until it reduces a little. When ready, top the turkey with gravy, and serve with a green side dish of your choice.

Spaghetti Squash Pasta

Serves 2

1 medium spaghetti squash	1 tablespoon pine nuts
2 cups diced crimini mushrooms	1 tablespoon olive oil
2 cups fresh basil	salt
1 tablespoon hemp seeds	pepper

Preheat the oven to 375°F. Put the squash in for thirty to forty minutes, until soft. When the shell of the squash is soft when poked with a fork, take it out of the oven, and cut it in half; let it cool, and with a spoon scoop the inside of the squash. Once you will start to pull it out the inside you will see the spaghetti like shape of the squash and you can put it in a plate to cool.

In a food processor, add the basil, hemp, pine nuts, salt, pepper, and olive oil; mix all together for the pesto. Clean and dice the mushrooms, and then cook them with a little olive oil, pepper, and salt in a pan until soft.

Set the spaghetti squash in a bowl, and mix it with some olive oil, pepper, and salt. Add it to the cooked mushrooms and sauté for two minutes. Finally add the pesto and serve. This is a great option for a gluten-free or vegan dinner.

Sautéed Coconut Carrots with Cod

Serves 4

3 large carrots	¼ cup capers
1½ tablespoons coconut oil	2 garlic cloves
¼ cup fresh oregano	olive oil
4 pieces cod	salt
2 large tomatoes	pepper
1 cup black olives	

Thinly slice the carrots in rounds, and set aside. Rinse the cod, and in a pan, add some olive oil and minced garlic. Add the cod, and sear it on both sides quickly. Toss in the cubed tomatoes, capers, and chopped black olives, and let it make a little sauce.

In another pan, mix the carrots with some water and coconut oil and cover; cook until soft. Then add the oregano. When the carrots are ready, set on the side of the cooked cod. Enjoy with a glass of white wine, if you want.

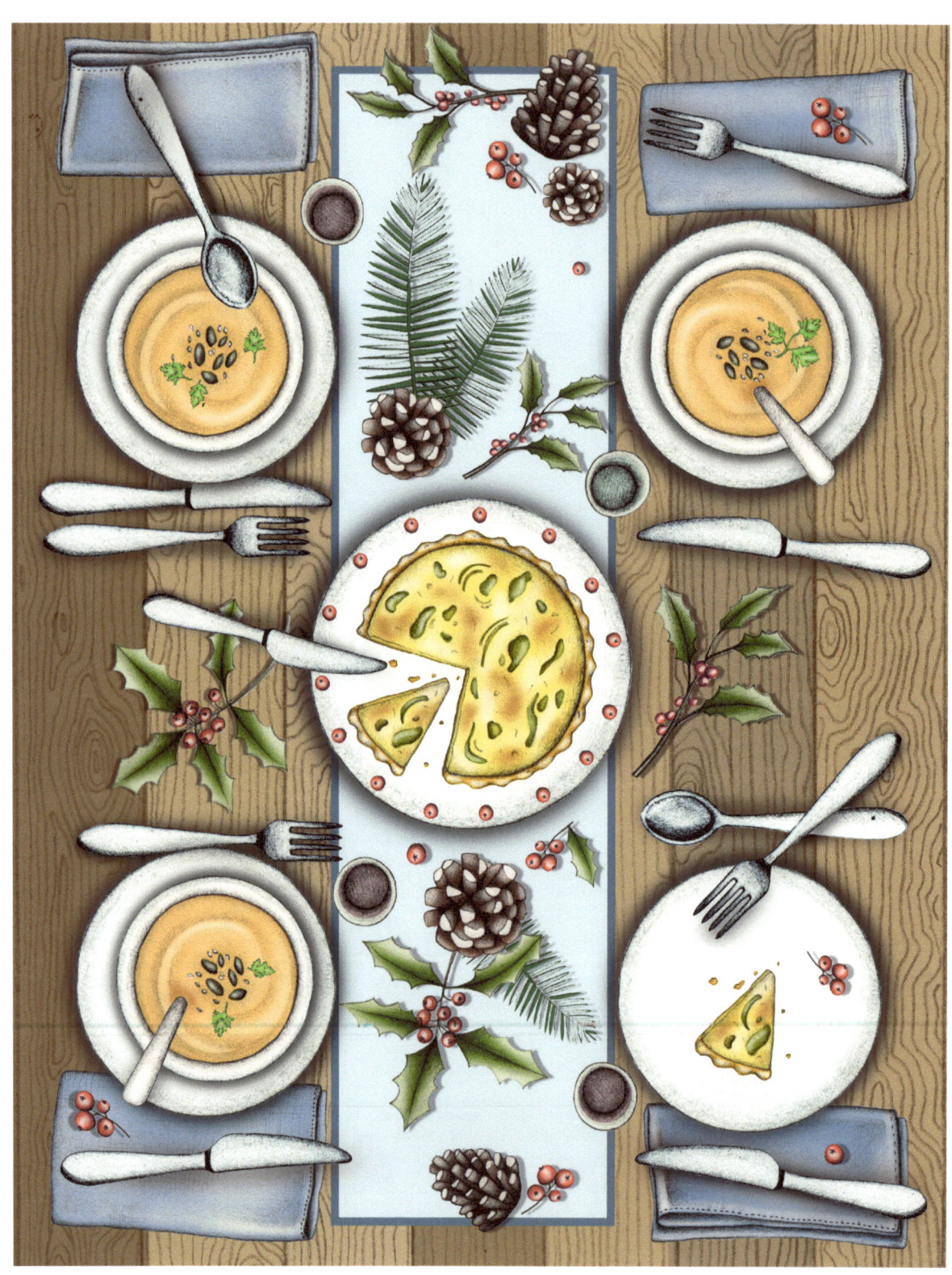

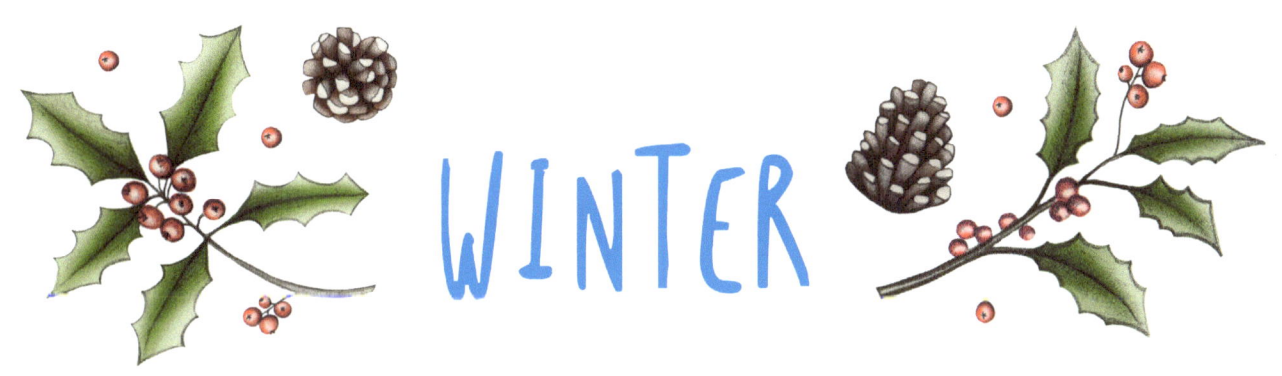

WINTER

Winter is that time of year where the earth offers us few choices, but this doesn't mean you can't make delicious food with seasonal ingredients. It's just a matter of a little more imagination.

In the winter food grows more slowly, which means vegetables keep more warmth in them—making them perfect for braising, roasting, or sautéing. At this time of year, you might want to add a little bit more protein and spices to warm yourself up.

Forward Fold (Uttanasana)

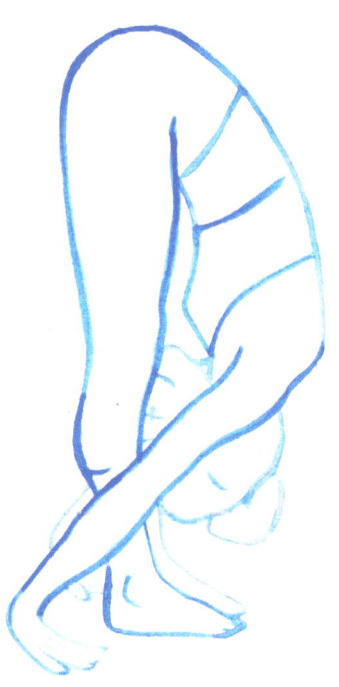

Winter in most countries means cold weather, when you will tend to stay inside and not see much light; you will move less and will tend to be a little more tired. Once in a while, take a few breaths and incorporate some movement so you don't feel too stiff.

Uttanasana is a great way to decompress you spine after sitting for long periods, to relax, and to let go. Make sure your feet are a little apart, knees microbent, and head loose, letting gravity take over. This position will help to open the shoulder joints, often strained from excessive typing, texting, or other small movements. It also exercises the colon, pancreas, and kidneys, which are extremely important organs for your internal well-being.

Breakfast

Buckwheat Pancakes

Serves 4

2 cups buckwheat flour
2 eggs
½ teaspoon baking soda
½ teaspoon cream of tartar or baking powder
almond milk, to mix
coconut oil, for cooking

Toppings:
cooked cinnamon apples or pears
maple syrup or honey
warmed blueberries

Mix all of the dry ingredients together; add the eggs and milk, and stir with a fork until the mixture is well combined. Heat up a pan, and add some coconut oil. Ladle the mixture into the pan to make medium-sized pancakes, and cook each side for a few minutes. Make sure the pan has enough coconut oil so that the pancakes do not stick. Serve warm with any toppings desired.

LUNCH

KABOCHA WINTER DETOX SOUP

Serves 4

1 medium kabocha squash	roasted sesame seeds, to taste
1 inch peeled ginger	sesame oil
2 garlic cloves	olive oil
1 teaspoon turmeric	homemade vegetable or bone broth
¼ teaspoon Himalayan salt	
1 handful cilantro	Foot note: More info for broths on page #58

Preheat the oven to 375°F. Put the squash in the oven for thirty minutes. When the squash is ready, put it aside to cool. Then cut it in half, remove the seeds and the green shell, and cut into pieces.

In a pot add garlic and sesame, and sauté for a few seconds. Add the squash, ginger, and turmeric; let it all cook for a few minutes, and then pour in the broth of your choice to cover everything. Let it cook for twenty minutes. If it boils, turn burner to low so it simmers. When all the ingredients are warm and feel soft, turn off the heat, and use a food processor to puree everything.

Serve warm with sesame seeds, cilantro, and a dash of olive oil on top.

KALE WITH BEETS AND MANDARIN SALAD

Serves 4

1 bunch kale	sesame oil
2 large beets	1 tablespoon miso
3 mandarin oranges	1 tablespoon mirin
2 tablespoons sliced almonds	2 handfuls of pumpkin seeds
1 tablespoon hemp	water, to mix
salt	

In a saucepan, add the beets with water to cover, put the lid on, and let boil for a minimum of thirty minutes, depending on their size. While the beets are cooking, cut the kale into pieces, and massage it a little to make it softer. Peel the mandarins, and toss it with the almonds and kale.

Poke the beets with a fork; if soft, they're ready. Place them in cold water; using gloves and a piece of paper towel, remove the skin and cut into small squares. Toss everything together, adding the hemp and pumpkin seeds. In a small bowl, mix the sesame oil, mirin, salt, miso, and water.

Serve the salad dressed.

LEEKS, CHARD, AND BACON QUICHE

Serves 6

For crust:

1 cup brown rice flour
¼ teaspoon baking powder

¼ teaspoon sea salt
1 large egg, slightly beaten
¼ cup butter, cut into small pieces
3 teaspoons cold water

For filling:
4 chard leaves
1 large leek
2 slices nitrite-free bacon
3 eggs

1 cup cashew milk
1 tablespoon mustard
salt
pepper
olive oil, to cook

Preheat the oven to 350°F. Make the crust first by adding flour, baking powder, and salt into a bowl. Add cold butter pieces, and use a fork to break. Add one egg and water, and stir until sticky. Roll dough out on a piece of waxed paper with rice flour on it. Turn the piece of waxed paper upside down into a pie pan. Note that the dough will not stick together like gluten dough. Bake for twenty-five to thirty minutes.

Rinse and then cut the leek as finely as possible. Finely chop the chard, and remove the stem form the leaves, as those cook by themselves faster. In a pan, cook the bacon until medium brown. Add some olive oil to another pan, and toss the leeks and chard stem; add some salt and a little bit of water, and cook for ten minutes. When everything is soft, add the chopped leaves, and cook for five more minutes. Remove from the heat and toss in a bowl with the other three eggs, milk, bacon pieces, pepper, salt, and mustard. Put everything in the pie crust.

Put the pie back in the oven, and let it cook for twenty to thirty minutes, or until the mixture is golden and hard. Enjoy warm with a salad on the side.

Snack

Sweet Potato Fries with Paleo "Mayo"

Serves 2

Fries:
1 large sweet potato
olive oil
salt

Sauce:
½ cup coconut cream, slightly warmed
½ cup warm water
¼ cup olive oil
3–4 garlic cloves
¼ teaspoon salt

Preheat the oven to 375°F. Cut the potatoes in slices as thin as you desire, set them in a baking sheet, and drizzle with olive oil and salt. Cook for thirty minutes. Meanwhile, make the sauce by warming the coconut cream and water and then adding the olive oil, garlic, and salt. Set in the fridge for fifteen minutes. When the potatoes are nicely cooked, serve with the sauce on the side.

Dinner

Portobello Burger

Serves 2

4 portobello mushroom caps
1 tablespoon coconut oil
2 medium slices halloumi cheese
¾ cup alfalfa sprouts

½ tablespoon mustard
1 teaspoon sauerkraut
1 teaspoon salt

Preheat the oven to 375°F. Wash the portobello mushrooms and slather the tops with coconut oil. Set them in an oven pan, and cook the mushrooms for fifteen minutes.

While they are cooking, take the halloumi and grill it.

When the mushroom are soft and brown, add the cheese, alfalfa, sauerkraut, and mustard, and enjoy warm!

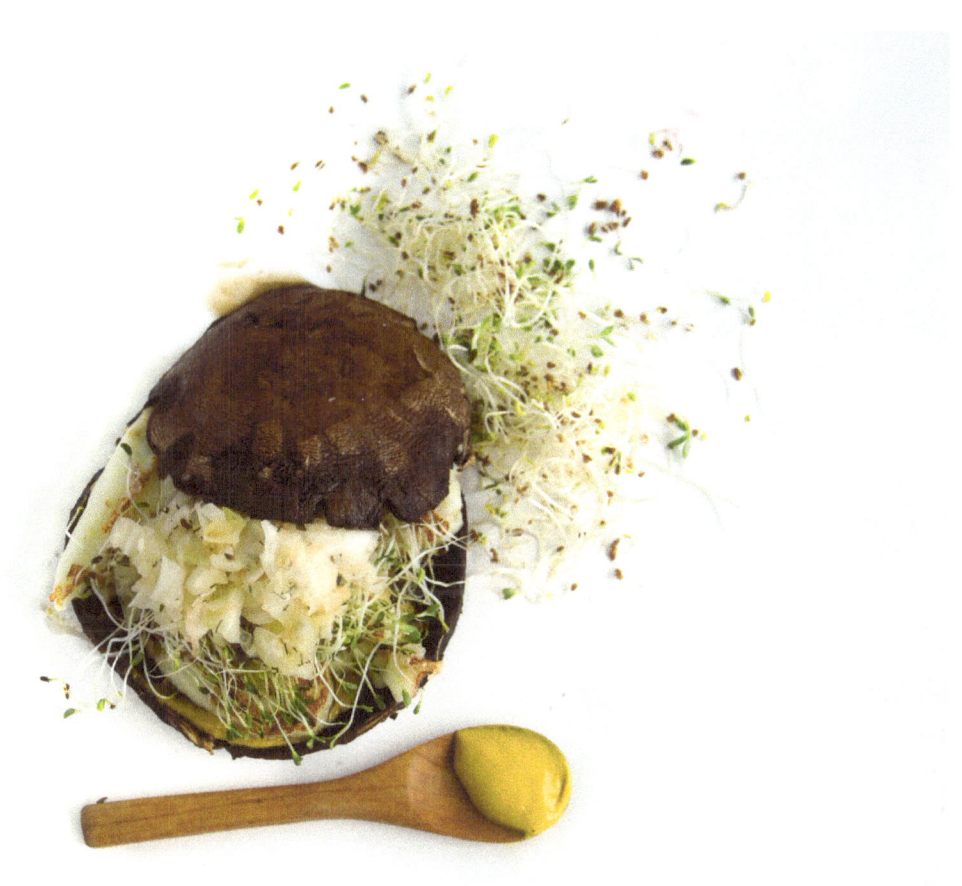

Potato and Chard Soup

Serves 2

For stock:	water, to fill	1 handful parsley
2 large carrots	salt	olive oil, to drizzle
1 large onion	For soup:	homemade vegetable
1 beet	2 cups organic russet potatoes	broth
4 celery stalks	1 bunch chard	

Add all of the vegetables to a large pot. Don't cut them unless they don't fit. Add water until everything is covered, and cook on low heat for two to three hours, until the stock reduces. Add salt almost at the end; the celery will release some saltiness while cooking. When ready, take the vegetables out, and set aside. You can serve them with olive oil, salt, and pepper. The broth can be kept up to four days in the fridge, or freeze it for future use.

Peel the potatoes, and set them in a bowl with lukewarm water so the starch releases for ten minutes. Then rinse them, cut into squares, and add them to the broth; boil for fifteen minutes. Add the chard and parsley afterward, and serve with a little olive oil drizzled on top.

Chicken alla Cacciatora

Serves 4

4 organic chicken thighs	1 tablespoon rosemary
1 onion	olive oil
1 cup red wine	salt
1 tablespoon thyme	pepper
1 tablespoon oregano	

Start by finely slicing the carrots with a mandolin, and set aside. Chop the onion as small as possible, and set aside.

Put some olive oil in a pan, and let it warm up a little. Rinse the thighs, and add them to the pan; sprinkle with salt and pepper. Let the thighs sauté for five minutes, browning each side. Mix all the spices together in a small bowl, top the chicken with it, and cook for another five minutes. The juices will release a little; add the wine and onion, cover, and cook on low heat for another ten to fifteen minutes. Open and poke the meat, or use a meat thermometer; the safe temperature for chicken is about 165°F. Serve warm with some sweet potatoes and leafy greens.

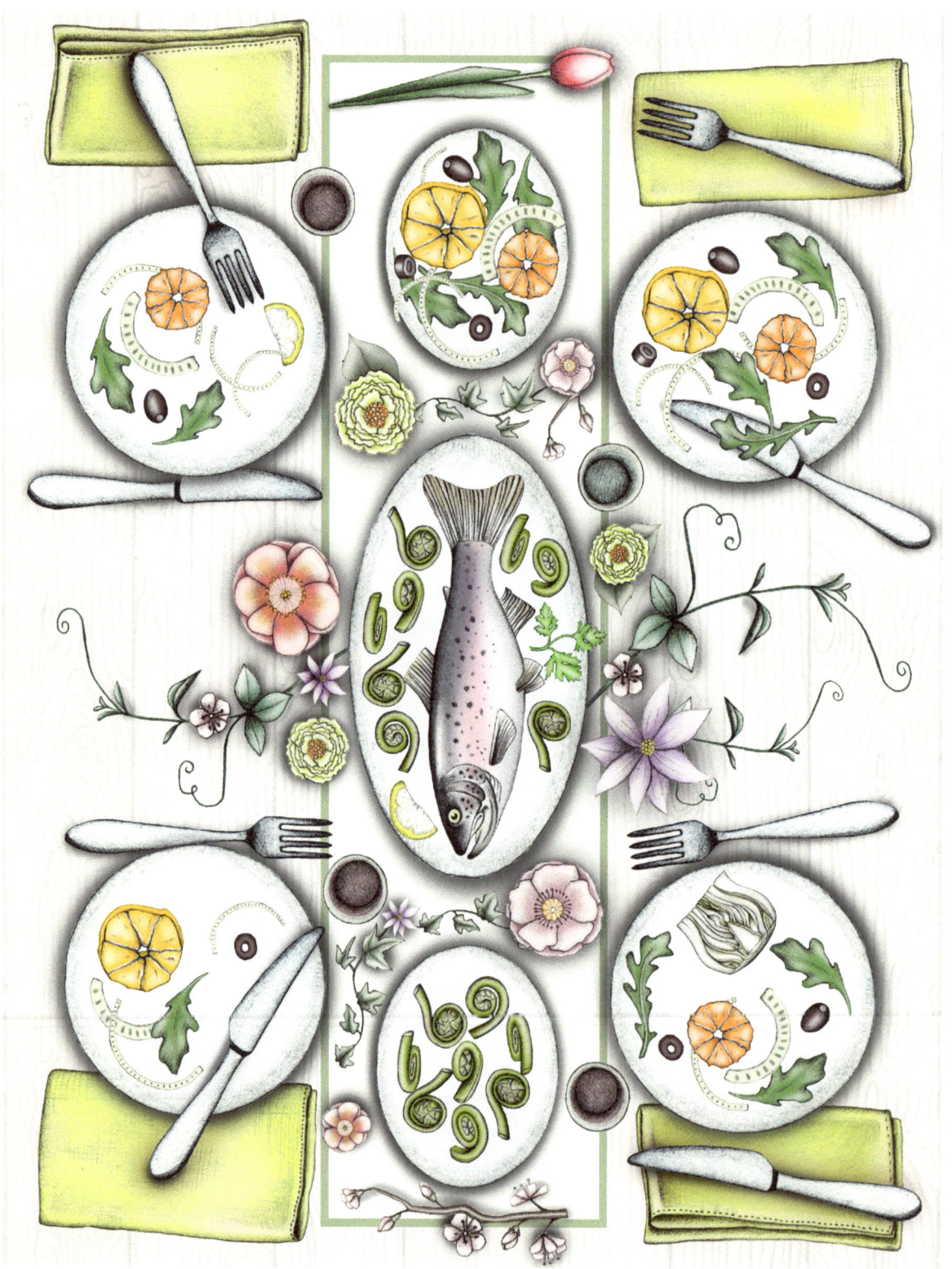

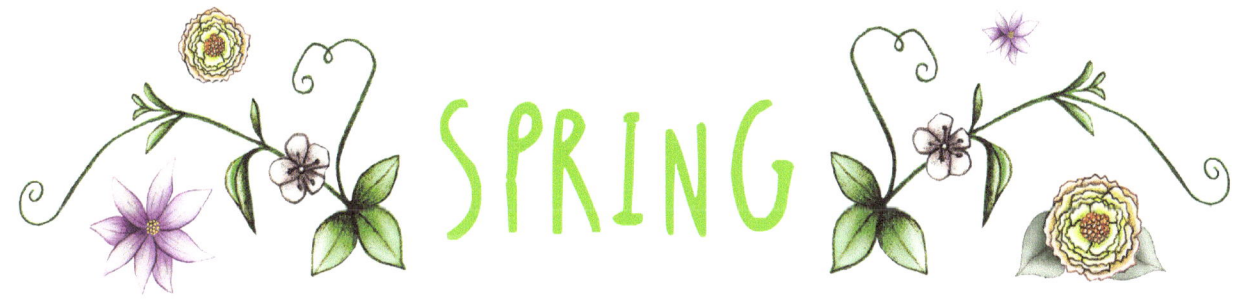

SPRING

Ah, spring—that time of year when the green is finally coming back, the flowers are blooming, and you feel more energized and full of life. I love spring because I can finally make my kitchen more colorful and enjoy the bountiful food mother earth offers us.

Color your table and plate with leafy greens to celebrate the rebirth of many vegetables. Grow your own herbs at this time of the year; it's fun and will give an extra zing to your plate.

TWISTED CHAIR (PARIVRTTA UTKATASANA)

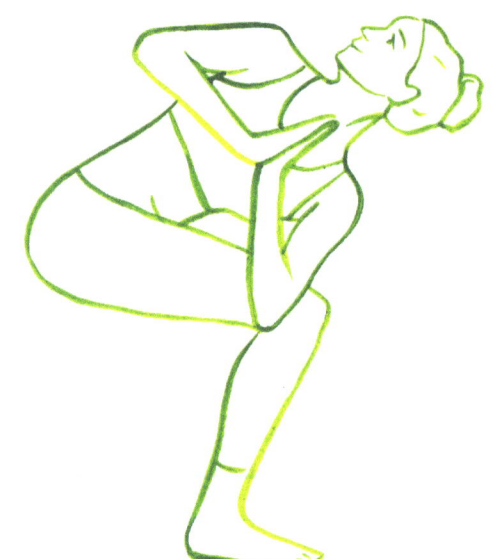

Spring is finally that season when you are ready to bloom again. It is a great time to detoxify and to cleanse from your body the stale toxins acquired during winter's time of limited movement.

With this position, you make your body strong by working the hip flexors, gluteus, and legs. With the twisting, you are able to detoxify your internal organs, focusing with stable breaths.

If this position needs modification, you can use a block or book between your thighs to increase your inner thighs' strength. If you feel your back can't round as much, avoid going too low. When twisting, also check that your knees are aligned.

BREAKFAST

GREEN SPRING DETOX SMOOTHIE

Serves 1

2 cups spinach
1 teaspoon turmeric
1 cup blueberries
1 cup cucumber
1 teaspoon maca

coconut water, to mix

Toppings:
sliced almonds
bee pollen

Mix all in a blender and serve topped with some sliced almonds and bee pollen. Chew your smoothie a little.

LUNCH

ZOODLE PASTA

Serves 2

2 medium zucchinis	Toppings:
2 garlic cloves, minced	pumpkin seeds
1 cup small tomatoes	parsley
1 tablespoon capers	
olive oil	
sesame oil	
salt	

With a spiralizer, make the zoodles; squeeze together to drain the extra water. In a pan, add the garlic to some sesame oil and warm up. Add the cut tomatoes and cook until soft; add the drained capers and cook. Mix in the zucchini and cook for a few minutes, until soft. Serve warm topped with pumpkin seeds and parsley.

EGGS WITH ASPARAGUS AND PROSCIUTTO

Serves 2

8 asparagus	olive oil
2 pasture-raised eggs	1 teaspoon ghee
8 slices organic La Quercia prosciutto	salt

Preheat the oven to 350°F. Rinse the asparagus and add to boiling water for ten minutes, until soft. Remove from the water and set in the oven for eight minutes. Remove from the oven again, and roll two or three asparagus in each slice of prosciutto. Return the asparagus to the oven, and cook another two minutes to crisp it up.

While the asparagus is cooking, make two eggs sunny-side up in a pan with the ghee. When the asparagus is ready, set on a plate, and add the egg on top. Plate with a salad on the side.

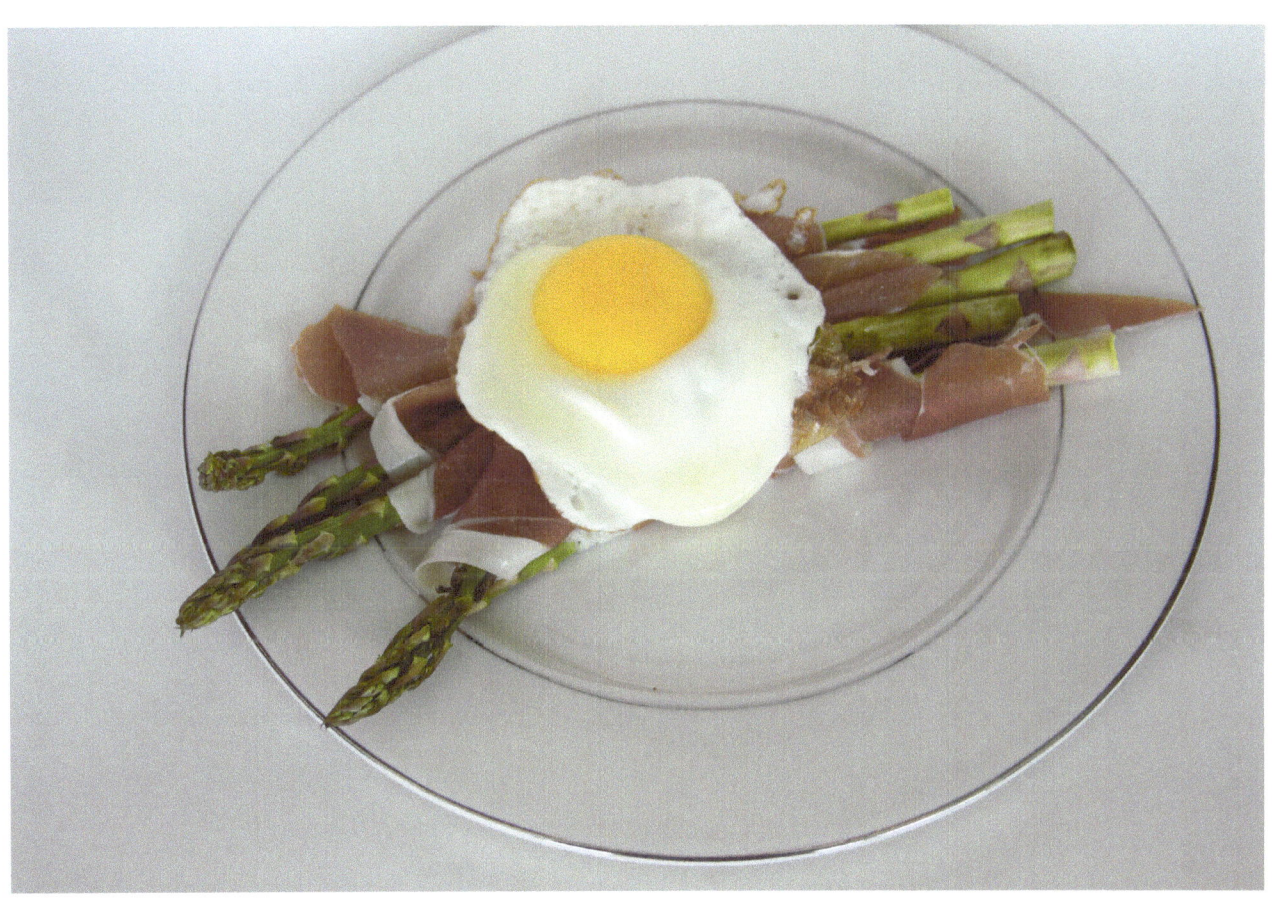

Arugula with Fennel and Orange Salad

Serves 4

4 handfuls arugula	2 tablespoons olive oil
1 large fennel	1 tablespoon balsamic vinegar
2 oranges	salt
1 handful pitted kalamata olives	pepper

Use a mandolin to slice the fennel. Drizzle with olive oil, salt, and vinegar, and mix it well. Add the arugula to the bottom of a serving bowl. Toss with the fennel, and then cover with olives and sliced oranges. Serve with a rice cake or a flaxseed cracker.

SNACK

Beet Hummus with Carrots

Serves 4

1 can BPA-free and kombu-soaked garbanzo beans	salt
	½ cup filtered water
1 large beet	1 handful parsley
1½ tablespoons tahini	olive oil
1½ lemons	½ cup water

Rinse and remove the liquid from the garbanzo beans. In a pot, cover the peeled beet with water and boil for twenty to thirty minutes, or until soft. Once cooled, slice the beet, and mix it with the beans in a food processor. Add tahini, salt, lemon, and parsley. Add one cup of olive oil and water to start, and pulse. Taste, and add a little more salt or parsley if needed.

You can eat this with carrots, celery, or black rice crackers.

DINNER

TROUT WITH FIDDLEHEADS

Serves 2

1 medium-fresh rainbow trout
olive oil
½ sliced lemon
1 bunch parsley

3 stems fresh thyme
salt
2 garlic cloves
3 cups fiddleheads

Preheat the oven to 350°F. Wash the fresh fish; add to its belly some lemon, salt, and half of the parsley and thyme. Enclose in foil and cook for twenty minutes.

Clean the fiddleheads, and set some olive oil and garlic to sauté in a pan. When the garlic is soft, toss in the fiddleheads with a little water and cook for ten to fifteen minutes more. When ready, cover with the rest of the parsley.

When everything is ready, serve one fillet of the trout on a plate with a side of vegetables. If you desire a glass of wine, a great match would be a Passerina or a Greco di Tufo.

SPRING PEA SOUP

Serves 2

6 cups fresh spring peas
2 cups homemade vegetable broth
1 large onion
½ cup coconut milk (optional homemade, in Chapter 8)

salt
1 small piece ginger
5–6 parsley stems
pepper
olive oil

Remove the peas from the shells, and set aside. Cut the onion and cook with some olive oil in a pot. When the onions are almost soft, add the peas and broth and cook for twenty to thirty minutes. When these are nice and soft, use a food processor or blender to mix the onion, broth, peas, and ginger; then add the coconut milk. Serve at room temperature with a drip of fresh olive oil and some parsley.

CAULIFLOWER RISOTTO

Serves 4

1 medium cauliflower
2 zucchinis
1 garlic clove
4 green onions
2 tablespoons sesame oil

1 cup collard greens or kale, finely chopped
1 teaspoon ginger
1 teaspoon tamari
1 cup parsley

With a blender, mince the cauliflower until it is fine and grainy. This might take a few rounds. In a pan, add the sesame oil, garlic, and green onions, and let them warm up a little; add the chopped zucchini and some salt, and keep mixing until the zucchini becomes golden and almost cooked. Lastly add the cauliflower and greens of your choice. Mix until everything is golden, and then add the tamari and parsley. Serve warm.

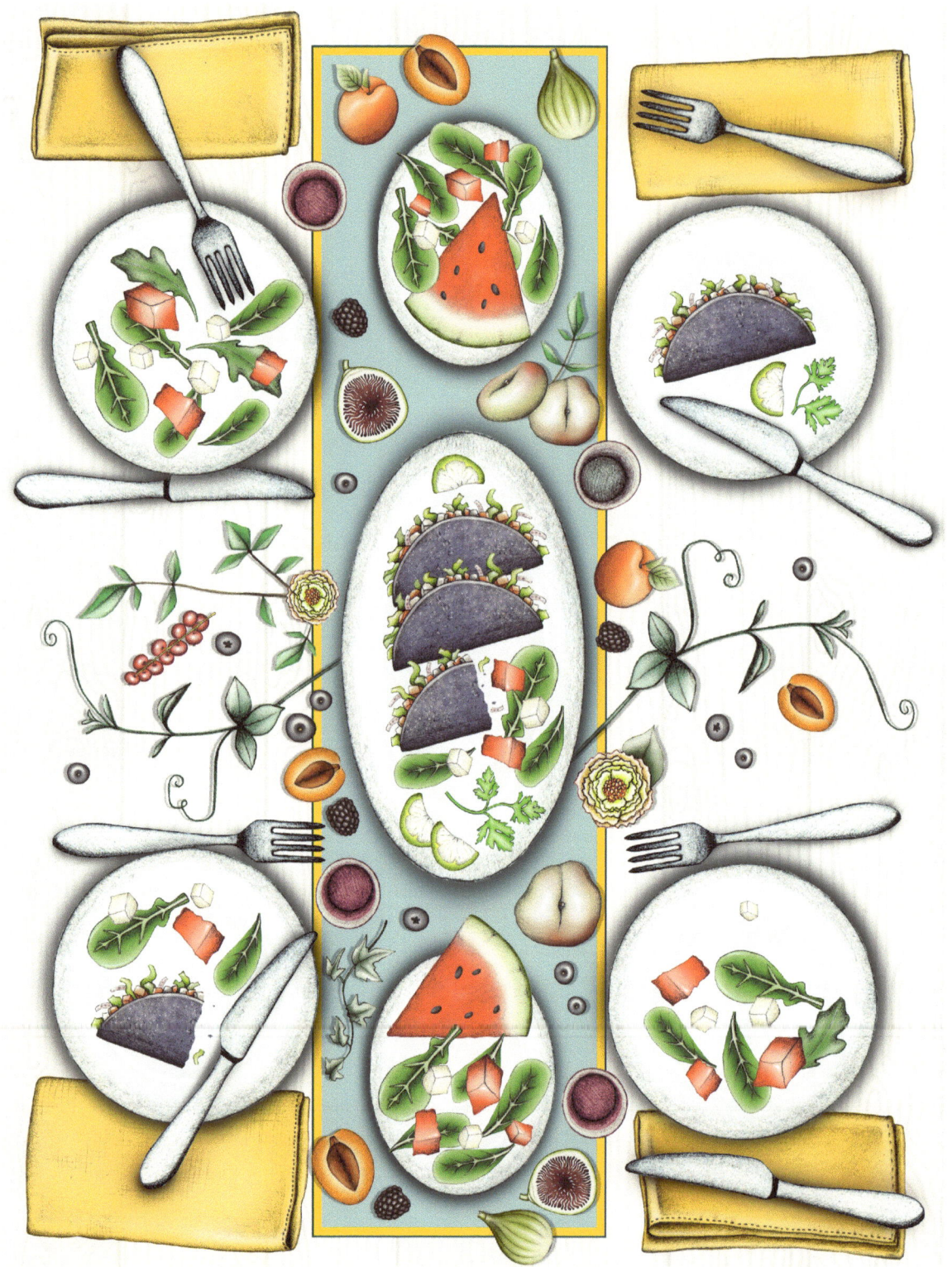

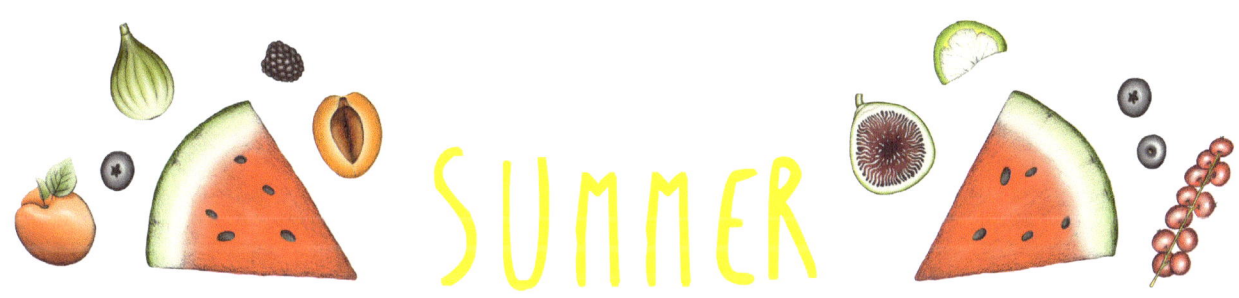

SUMMER

Summer is that time of year where the sun is warm; you might enjoy a vacation, the beach, barbecues, and family time, and fill your plates with juicy fruits and a rainbow-colored salad. This season takes me back to my days boating; getting fresh fish caught from the local fish co-operative; and snacking on juicy peaches, apricots, and all of summer's delicious foods.

This time of year, if it's really warm, you get less hungry, so stick with cooling and light foods, as those in Chinese medicine would say. Love the many colors in the fruits and vegetables, using cilantro or peppermint to add flavor.

SUPPORTED SHOULDER STAND (SARVANGASANA)

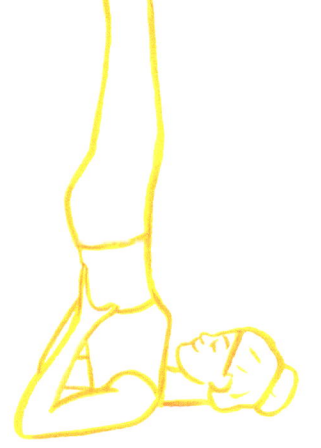

In the summer we feel we have tons of energy, and we are surrounded by warmth and colors. Your body needs some cooling, and with the supported shoulder stand, you will be able to get that feeling.

With this position, you will be able to improve many organs and muscles, such as your digestive tract, due to the change in gravity and by stimulating the thyroid and circulation and oxygenizing the lungs. Your heart will thank you, because it needs to do less work to pump the blood around.

If you have neck issues, try to use a blanket under the shoulders. Count about three fingers between your shoulders and the end of the blanket, making sure the neck is relaxed and gives a little more space to your neck. Stay in this position, if possible, for a minimum of one minute or up to fifteen minutes.

Breakfast

Summer Chia Seed Pudding

Serves 1

½ cup peaches, peeled and cubed
1 cup raspberries
1 teaspoon lemon

¼ cup chia seeds
1 cup homemade coconut milk

Mix the chia seeds with the milk, and set aside. In a pot, add the raspberries and peaches with the lemon, and let it warm up at a low heat. If needed, add one tablespoon of filtered water. Cook until it becomes a little compote.

When the chia seeds are all puffed up and look gelatinous, top with the fruits. Enjoy with a cup of your favorite tea or coffee, and you will feel energized and full until lunch.

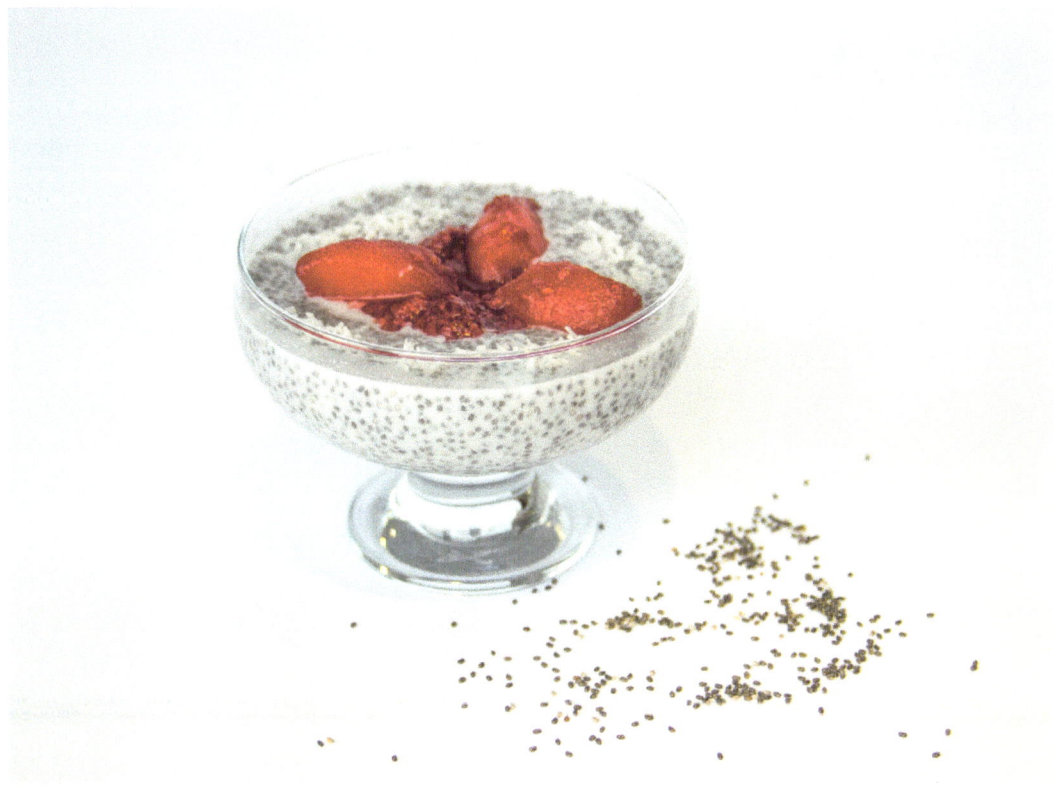

LUNCH

SUMMER ROLL

Serves 2

2 rainbow carrots	Sauce:
1 bunch cilantro	¼ cup almond butter
1 cucumber	1 tablespoon liquid aminos
1 handful alfalfa sprouts (make your own)	1 tablespoon rice vinegar
1 medium beet	1 tablespoon water
4 rice papers	½ inch piece peeled ginger
water to soften the paper sheets	

To make the alfalfa sprouts, set one tablespoon alfalfa seeds in a jar and cover with water. Leave overnight. The morning after, take a cheesecloth and a rubber band, cover the top of the jar with the cloth, and rinse the alfalfa. Do this two times a day for five days, and the sprouts will be ready. The more you keep rinsing them, the more they grow.

Set the beet in a pot; cover it with water and boil for twenty minutes. Slice the carrots and cucumber, and wash the sprouts and cilantro.

Mix all the wet ingredients for the sauce in a pan, and grate the ginger; mix for three to four minutes until everything is nice and smooth.

When the beet is soft and cool, peel and slice it. Take a plate with high rims and fill with water. Place one sheet of rice paper in it to make it softer; soak for six seconds. Use another plate to set the soft paper on, and fill up the soft paper with all the vegetables and sprouts. Roll everything. Be gentle and make sure no vegetable has a sharp edge or the paper will break. Repeat until the four rolls are done. These are great treats for a party, a date night, or a light dinner.

Spinach, Feta, and Watermelon Salad

Serves 4

3 cups fresh baby spinach	lemon
¼ watermelon (or ½ small one)	olive oil
1½ cups cubed feta	salt
balsamic vinegar	

Toss the spinach and feta together. Cube the watermelon, and add to the serving bowl. In a different bowl, make the dressing with the wet ingredients. Pour over the salad. This recipe is simple, easy, and refreshing.

Rainbow Summer Salad

Serves 2

1 cup watercress	8 shrimps
1 cup microgreens	sesame oil
2 seasonal tomatoes	olive oil
2 rainbow carrots	salt
1 tablespoon hemp seeds	balsamic vinegar
1 tablespoon sliced almonds	lemon

Mix all the greens with the hemp and almonds. In a pan, cook the shrimp with a little sesame oil and salt for only three minutes. When ready, take them out and set on the salad. In a small bowl, mix olive oil, salt, lemon, and balsamic vinegar, and pour the mix on the salad.

SNACK

STRAWBERRY, MICROGREEN AND FARMER'S CHEESE

Serves 2

4 strawberries
1 spoon farmer cheese
1/2 spoon balsamic vinegar
Salt
Microgreen to top

Quart the strawberries, mix the cheese and add the vinegar and salt. Top with the microgreen and enjot this fresh snack on a warm summer day.

DINNER

SARDINES

Serves 2

8 sardines   ½ cup small tomatoes
1 cup parsley   olive oil
bread crumbs or almond meal (gluten-free choice)   salt

Preheat the oven to 375°F. Rinse the sardines, and set in an oven pan. In a bowl mix the crumbs of choice with the salt, a little olive oil, and minced parsley. Cover the sardines with the bread mixture, and mix in the tomatoes cut in halves. Cook in the oven for fifteen minutes. Serve warm with a salad on the side.

LAMB SKEWERS AND GRILLED VEGGIES

Serves 2

16 cubed pieces of lamb	Vegetables:
3 cup mineral water	2 zucchini
2 mint stems	2 medium onions
½ cup olive oil	1 eggplant
salt	1 handful parsley
pepper	1 tablespoon lemon
skewers	1 teaspoon salt
	¼ cup olive oil

Set the lamb in the mineral water with some salt, and let it rest for at least one hour. Cut the mint and mix with the rest of the ingredients, and set aside. Cut the vegetables in slices that are one inch thick. Make a mixture of olive oil, salt, and pepper in another bowl, and add some of the trimmed parsley. Bathe the vegetables with half the mixture and use the other half for the meat.

When the meat has marinated for some time, put it on the skewers, top with the mixture, and start cooking. Grill until tender on each side. If you have a meat thermometer, check the temperature; lamb should be 145°F for a medium-rare skewer.

You will cook the vegetables first, and then set the mixture on top, and let the dish sit a few minutes before serving. This is a great summer recipe to do at a barbecue. You can accompany it with a summer salad, some local corn on the cob, and some homemade fruit water.

FISH BLUE-CORN TACOS

Serves 2

2 wild cod fillets	3 small tomatoes
1 handful cilantro	¼ jicama
1 lime	1 small onion
4 blue-corn tortillas	olive oil
½ avocado	salt

Cook the cod in a pan with a little olive oil and salt for four minutes. Set aside. In the same pan, sauté the onion. Chop the avocado, and mash with a fork. Add the tomatoes, cubed as small as possible. Shred the jicama, and chop the cilantro. Set aside.

In the tortilla, put the fish first and then cover with the avocado, a spritz of lime, the sautéed onions, jicama, and cilantro. Here is a fresh and filling dinner that can be accompanied with a summer salad or some black rice.

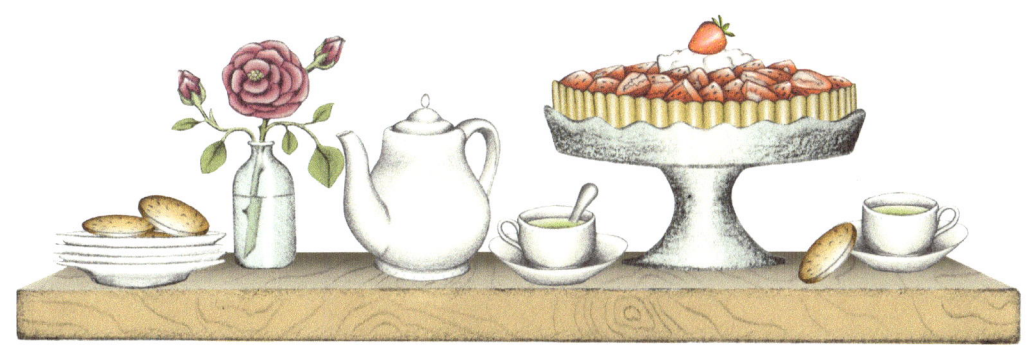

CHAPTER 7
Dessert

• • •

Sugar today is becoming a big enemy, and it is a key contributor to many of the diseases the United States faces, such as obesity and type 2 diabetes—which means that you want to stay away from packaged cookies, cakes, and hidden sugars. I decided to add this section because all of us have that sweet tooth. But you can have a dessert that tastes good without compromising your body.

Fall: Apple Orange Crumble

Serves 6

1 apple	2 tablespoons coconut oil
1 large orange	1 cup coconut sugar
1½ cups almond flour	1 tablespoon pine nuts
1 cup rolled oats	

Preheat the oven to 350°F. Peel and slice the apple, and peel the orange. Set every slice on a cookie sheet. In a bowl, mix the almond flour, oats, coconut oil, sugar, and pine nuts. Top the fruit with this mixture and cook for twenty minutes, until the top is browned. Serve with some coconut cream or ice cream.

Coconut Cream:
1 BPA-free coconut milk can
1 tablespoon coconut sugar

Set the can in the fridge for at least one hour. Open the can; make sure to not shake it. With a spoon, scoop out the top part which it became solid, and put it in a cake mixer. Add the sugar. Whip for five minutes, until smooth. Set in the fridge for ten minutes if you want it to be a little less runny.

Winter: Ginger Tea Cookies

Serves 6

2¼ cups almond meal	1½ teaspoons baking powder
2 tablespoons coconut sugar	3 tablespoons coconut oil
1 teaspoon cinnamon	2 tablespoons blackstrap molasses
2½ teaspoons ground ginger	3 teaspoons vanilla extract
½ teaspoon sea salt	2 tablespoons coconut nectar or honey
1½ teaspoons baking soda	

Preheat the oven to 350°F. Mix together the almond meal, baking soda, baking powder, spices, salt, and sugar in a bowl. In a small saucepan, melt the coconut oil. In another bowl, mix the molasses, vanilla extract, and coconut syrup or honey. Add the oil to the liquids, and then pour the liquids into the center of the dry ingredients. Mix well, and taste to make sure it's sweet enough. Spoon into a cookie form on a baking sheet lined with parchment paper. Set the sheet in the oven to cook for ten to twelve minutes. When the cookies are browned, set them to cool outside, and then place them in a cookie jar to eat later with your tea, coffee, or as a sweet treat.

SPRING: CHOCOLATE APRICOT CAKE

Serves 8

3 apricots
2 cups almond flour
1 egg
1 teaspoon baking soda
½ teaspoon baking powder

½ cup almond milk
1 cup coconut milk from can
4 tablespoons raw cocoa powder
1 cup coconut syrup, divided

Coconut milk instructions: The night before, set the coconut milk can in the fridge. The day of, open the can, making sure to not shake it, and remove only the top part (the cream) for the icing.

Preheat the oven to 375°F. Mix the almond flour, baking powder, and baking soda together in a bowl; add the egg and almond milk. Make sure you get a liquid consistency.

Clean and cut the peaches in cubes, and toss them in the mixture. Add ½ cup coconut syrup, taste, and adjust for sweetness. Pour into a baking cake pan, and cook for thirty minutes. To check if ready, use a toothpick and dip it in the middle of the cake; if it's liquid it's not ready and you will cook for ten more minutes.

As the cake cooks, add the coconut milk, cocoa powder, and the other ½ cup of coconut syrup to a saucepan, and mix until combined. Set in the fridge for fifteen minutes to solidify.

When the cake is ready, let it cool, and then add the frosting. This is a delicious treat for dessert with family or friends. If you prefer not too much of a sweet taste, reduce the amount of sweetener for the cake, as the frosting will keep it sweet.

SUMMER: STRAWBERRY PIE WITH COCONUT CREAM

Crust:
½ cup coconut oil, melted
4 eggs
½ teaspoon salt
1 cup coconut flour
4 tablespoons raw honey

Filling:
2 pounds strawberries
2 tablespoons raw honey
juice of ½ lemon
½ tablespoon arrowroot powder

Cream:
1 BPA-free can of coconut milk
2 tablespoons coconut nectar or sweetener of choice

Preheat the oven to 400°F. Set the coconut can in the fridge. First make the crust by mixing the flour, honey, and salt. Melt the coconut oil in a small saucepan, and pour it into the flour mixture. Add the eggs, and mix everything until it becomes a nice ball. Set it in the baking pan you will use. Pat down to make it as even as possible. Cook for nine to ten minutes, checking on it so it doesn't burn.

In another saucepan, add half cup of finely chopped strawberries, lemon, and honey, and let it cook at a medium heat. Stir it often to make sure it doesn't burn. After it has cooked for about eight minutes, add the arrowroot powder, and stir to mix well. Remove from heat, and let it cool.

Chop the rest of the strawberries as small as possible, and put them in a bowl. Add in the strawberry and lemon mixture, and stir well. Set the bowl in the fridge for one hour.

After an hour, take the strawberries out and pour on top of the crust. Preheat the oven to 350°F, and then cook for ten to fifteen minutes to soften the fruit. Take out, and let it cool.

While the cake cooks, take the can of coconut milk out, and remove only the solid white part of the coconut milk. Add this to a bowl, and let it sit for ten minutes to get to room temperature. Then beat it with an electric beater. Pour your sweetener of choice in, and mix it well until you get a creamy texture. Set aside.

Serve the cake cut into triangles and topped with cream. You will impress everyone with this delicious and healthy dessert.

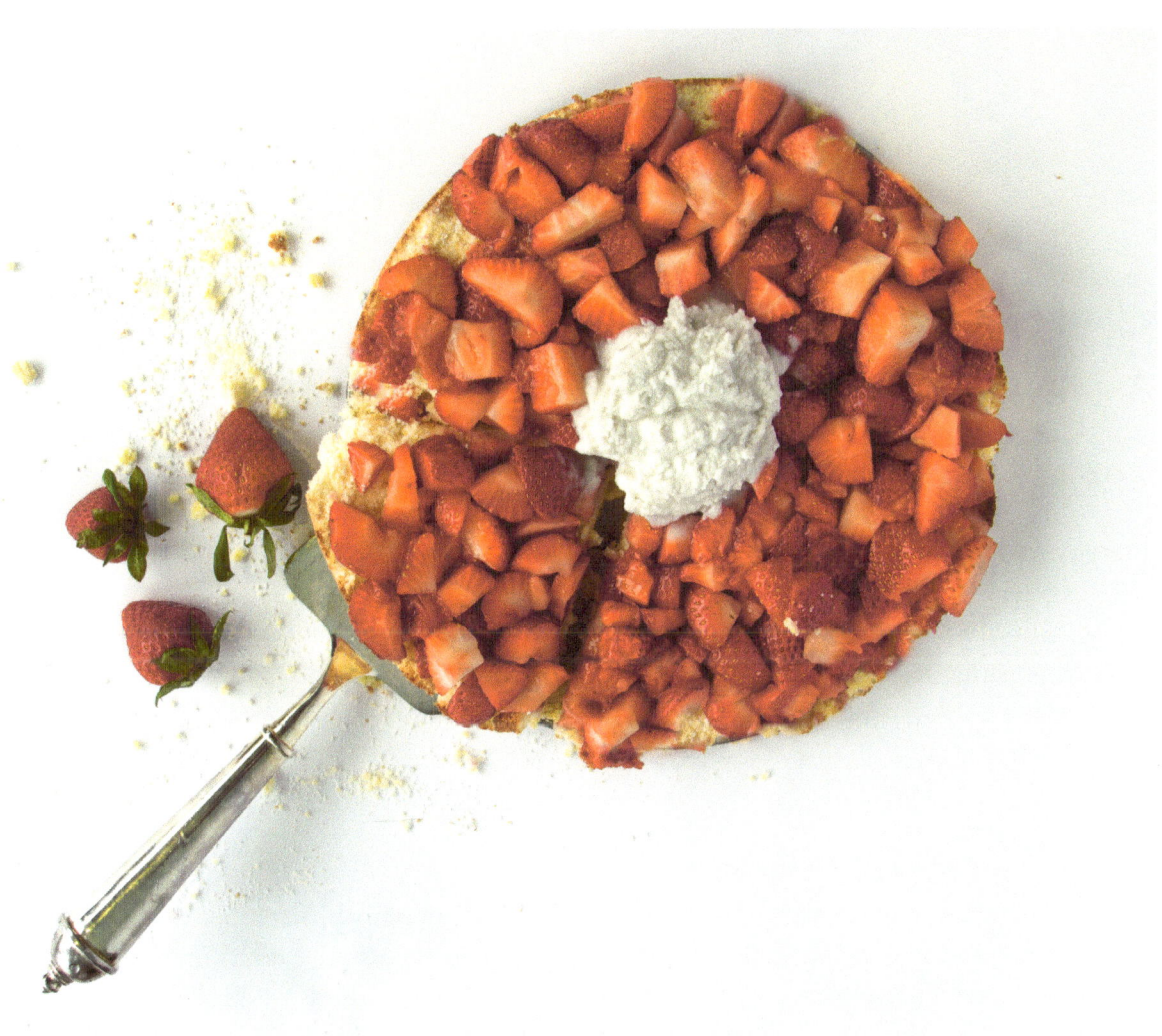

CHAPTER 8
Broths and Milks

• • •

ARIANNA'S HOMEMADE VEGETABLE BROTH

Serves 6

1 large carrot
3 stalks celery
1 large beet
1 bunch of parley
1 large onion
1 sweet potato
salt
water to cover

Peel the onion, toss all the vegetables in a large pot, and cover with water. Set the heat at medium and bring to boil. Then lower the heat, and cover. Let it cook for four to five hours minimum, until the stock reduces. Add salt almost at the end; the celery will release some saltiness while cooking. Then remove the vegetables and use the broth. When ready, remove the vegetables. (Sometimes I just take out the carrots, potato, and beet, and eat them with some olive oil and salt to avoid throwing them out.) The broth can be kept up to four days in the fridge, or freeze it for future use.

Homemade Chicken-Bone Broth

Serves 6

1 chicken carcass
1 onion
3 stalks celery
1 large carrot
1 parsley bunch
1 inch ginger
salt
water to cover

Peel the onion, toss all the vegetables in a large pot with the chicken, and cover with water. Set the heat at medium and bring to boil. Then lower the heat and cover. Let it cook for ten to twelve hours or until the stock reduces. Once in a while, open the pot, and remove the brown curd you will get from the bones. Add salt almost at the end; the celery will release some saltiness while cooking. When ready the carcass will be all softened and breaking up; remove, and if there is some meat on it remove from bone and keep in the broth. Remove the vegetables. Pour the broth in a jar, and use when needed for other recipes or soups.

Homemade Superfast Coconut Milk

Serves 6

2 cups coconut (shredded, unsweetened)
2 dates (optional for sweetness)
4 cups water
1 tablespoon vanilla powder

Add coconut, vanilla, and water in a blender. If you want to add the dates, make sure they are pitted. Blend for three minutes, and then, with a cheesecloth separate, the liquid from the solid part. Keep in the fridge up to three days. Use for coffee, soups, teas, breakfast oatmeal, and more.

At-Home Almond Milk

Serves 4

2 cups peeled almonds
6 cups water
2 dates
1 tablespoon vanilla powder
2 tablespoon cocoa (if you want to make it for children)
1 tablespoon turmeric (for a detox milk)

Soak the almonds in water; set on the fridge overnight. The day after, rinse them, and put them in the blender with the dates and vanilla or optional cocoa, turmeric. Blend for five minutes or so; add water if the mixture is still thick. With a nut bag or cheesecloth, separate the solid from the liquid. Put it in a glass jar with a sealed top, and put in the fridge for up to four days. Use for coffee, soups, teas, breakfast oatmeal, and more.

Acknowledgments

. . .

I WANT TO THANK THE people who have helped me achieve this goal:

My husband, who has always believed in me and stood by my side. His support and enthusiasm pushed me to make this happen.

My sister, who gave me the idea and courage to write this book.

My mother, who taught me to cook, to listen to myself, and to understand who I am. With this skill, I have put in practice my passions and have become an author of this first book.

Tilla, who made the beautiful illustrations for this book and who was able to convey my messages with simplicity and love.

About the Author

• • •

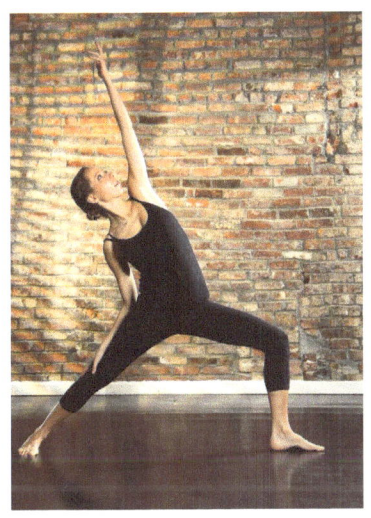

ARIANNA IS A HOLISTIC HEALTH coach who graduated from the Institute for Integrative Nutrition in 2013. She is also a yoga teacher who trained both at Yoga Works and Bend & Bloom in New York City. She is a self trained chef that cooks for New York families, events and teaches private classes. After her training, her life changed when she realized that cooking and teaching people how to eat and move were her passions and were areas in which she wanted to expand her knowledge. In 2015 she founded her LLC and website Feed the Body and Soul, and she's deeply passionate about inspiring people to embrace change and to feel better.

www.ingramcontent.com/pod-product-compliance
Lightning Source LLC
Chambersburg PA
CBHW060832290526
45792CB00006BB/1895